14 Days to a Healthier You

A Complete Guide to Effective Weight Loss

By
Amber Rose

Table of Contents

<u>Workout Plans</u>

<u>Recipes Plan and Ideas</u>

Introduction

Welcome to "14 Days to a Healthier You: A Complete Guide to Effective Weight Loss." The likelihood is that if you choose to read this book, you are seeking to improve your health and well-being and make good changes in your life. You've made an important first step, and I applaud your dedication to bettering yourself.

It's simple to become perplexed and upset when it comes to weight reduction in a society full of fad diets, fast fixes, and an abundance of contradictory advice. This book strives to cut through the clutter and provide you with a straightforward, scientifically supported, and doable plan for losing those excess pounds and leading a healthy lifestyle.

The 14-day period we'll be emphasizing is not about predicting magical changes, but rather about launching your weight reduction journey and putting you on the road to long-lasting outcomes. You will discover the foundations of successful weight reduction during these two weeks, including appropriate diet, exercise, mentality, and lifestyle modifications.

This book is intended to assist you in achieving your goals, whether you want to lose weight specifically, increase your energy, or just feel better about yourself. It's about making long-term decisions that will be good for your health and mind, not about drastic tactics like crash diets.

You may discover helpful recommendations, doable actions, example food plans, exercise routines, and assistance for sustaining your improvement beyond the first 14 days in the pages that follow. We'll look at the science of weight reduction, motivation psychology, and the significance of creating enduring habits.

Keep in mind that every person's road to losing weight is different, and your outcomes may vary. The secret is to approach this trip with patience, perseverance, and a desire to learn, and to put the emphasis on progress rather than perfection.

Are you thus prepared to change your life in only 14 days? Together, let's take this trip to learn how you may transform into a healthier, happier version of yourself. Your journey to a healthy you starts right now.

Understanding Weight Loss

Calories factor into the equation while trying to maintain a healthy weight. The key to losing weight is to burn more calories than you consume. You may do this by consuming fewer calories than you need and increasing the number of calories you burn via physical exercise.

Even though it appears straightforward, putting into practice a sensible, efficient, and lasting weight-loss strategy may be difficult.

You don't have to do it alone, however. For assistance, consult your physician, your family, and your friends. Consider if this is the right moment and whether you're prepared to make the essential adjustments. Plan wisely as well: Consider how you'll respond to circumstances that put your determination to the test and the inevitable slight setbacks.

Your doctor can recommend weight-loss surgery or drugs for you if you are very overweight and experiencing health issues. In this situation, your doctor will go through the potential advantages and hazards with you.

But keep in mind that changing your eating and activity habits is essential if you want to lose weight successfully.

Setting Goals

Many fad diets, weight-reduction plans, and outright frauds promise effortless and speedy weight loss. The cornerstone of effective weight reduction, however, continues to be a wholesome, calorie-restricted diet together with increased physical activity. You must make long-lasting adjustments to your eating habits and way of life if you want to lose weight successfully and permanently.

Setting realistic weight-loss targets can seem intuitive. But are you aware of what is realistic? Aiming to lose 1 to 2 pounds (0.5 to 1 kilogram) every week is a wise long-term strategy.

Typically, you need to burn 500–1,000 more calories per day than you take in via a reduced-calorie diet and consistent exercise to lose 1–2 pounds each week.

Depending on your weight, losing 5% of it could be a feasible objective, at least initially. 9 pounds (4 kilograms) is the equivalent of 82 kilograms (180 pounds) in weight. Your chance of developing chronic health conditions like heart disease and type 2 diabetes may be decreased with even this degree of weight reduction.

Consider both process and end goals while establishing your objectives. Process goals include things like "Walk for 30 minutes every day." The outcome objective "lose 10 pounds" is an illustration of this. Although it is not necessary to have an end objective, it is advisable to have process goals since altering your behaviors is the key to losing weight.

The Science of Weight Loss

Because of how the body reacts to weight reduction, it may be challenging to lose weight and keep it off: The body makes an effort to regain any lost weight. It's crucial to eat healthily and move more, but for many individuals, these strategies may not be sufficient to maintain weight loss.

It is real. Hormones that originate from various bodily regions, such as the stomach, intestines, and adipose tissue, send messages about hunger to the neurological system, which includes the brain, throughout the day. What, why, and how much we eat is influenced by both the brain and these appetite hormones.

In other cases, even when we don't need it, our brain reacts to hunger hormones by telling us we need to get some.

Other times, even though we are not hungry, our brain may send signals that make us want to eat for pleasure.

The brain determines how to respond to impulses like hunger, pleasure, and other emotions.

Chapter 1

Setting the Foundation

Food is used for much more than simply providing energy for our bodies in society and daily life. It is present in practically all of our activities. Everything is edible!

Along with providing nutrition for our bodies, eating serves a multitude of other purposes. It is relational, social, cultural, and emotional. I'll be the first to say that I have eaten just because the food was placed in front of me at a party or social event when I was feeling down or anxious, or simply because I was hungry. We develop so many of our dietary habits unconsciously.

Despite the food-obsessed world we now inhabit, it is feasible to alter your diet, eat healthier food, feel better physically, and shed some pounds. It just requires a little amount of foresight, planning, and preparation. If you want to regain control over your food and create healthy habits for life, laying a solid foundation for weight reduction is essential.

Setting precise objectives will result in considerably more productivity. Consider setting a deadline for completing a specific distance of running or signing up for a race or athletic event. Regular (daily) exercise to prepare for the event and an improvement in your nutrition to ensure your body performs at its best are the practical measures to reach this aim. Weight reduction is a benefit of maintaining a regular exercise routine and a balanced diet to help you reach your goal.

A step back from the food, nutrition, calories, and preparation might often be all that is necessary to see the greater picture. Food is not the only thing that matters in life. Consider it a tool to assist you in living properly.

Meal planning

If I could offer you just one piece of advice to help you eat healthier and lose weight, it would be this: "Plan your family's meals every week, write your shopping list at the same time, and only buy the items on your list."

Meal planning accomplishes two goals.

- It will specify what is given at each meal for you. By doing this, you may avoid worrying about what to bring for lunch when you wake up in the morning or about supper each evening as you drive home from work.
- You'll have everything you need to prepare the meals on the menu since you've created a shopping list based on your meal plan. Making fewer visits to the store can help you save a tonne of money.

Burn Body Fat

The kind of food you consume has a huge impact on whether your body is burning fat or storing it. The complicated interplay of chemicals, hormones, enzymes, and the kinds of foods and nutrients we ingest affects both metabolism and fat accumulation. Dietary strategies that trigger the body to start burning fat and lose weight are a crucial component of any effective weight reduction program. Losing weight that is made up of fluid or muscle is useless. We want the body to start burning stored body fat since it's what causes the health issues that come with being overweight.

To successfully lose weight over the long run, one must choose foods that are rich in fiber, good quality carbs, low-fat proteins, and healthy fats. A large diet of fresh vegetables and two servings of fruit are equally crucial. If we want to keep our hunger under control, feel fuller for longer, have excellent nutritional and digestive health, and most importantly, get our body burning fat, we must always include these elements in every meal.

Bringing Everything Together

Everything ultimately boils down to what you put in your mouth. Even if you are a nutrition expert, it won't help your family eat well if you don't have the tools and expertise to make it happen. I like demonstrating to others how simple it is to make fast, wholesome meals that the whole family will enjoy.

Start arming yourself with the skills to translate your nutrition knowledge into a nutritious dinner on your plate if you're serious about attaining long-term weight reduction and excellent health. Planning, shopping, cooking, and serving meals are essential skills for long-term healthy eating.

Clearing Out Your Pantry

There is a link between your weight, health, and the food you keep in your pantry, which is a little-known fact. It's the same as keeping things beneath your bed to keep cookies, nutritionally-deficient crackers, cans of crappy soup, and the unopened bag of white flour on the shelf. Even though you don't always see it, you are aware that it exists.

- Stress is produced.

- It leads to compulsive thinking (e.g.: "Oh, there are cookies in the cabinet").
- Every time you open the cupboard, mental clutter results (I need to clear out this cabinet.

Here are 8 ways to revamp the shelves in your pantry:

1. Throw Out Apparent "Junk" Food: Unless it's something you love and incorporate into your diet with healthy choices, Get. Rid. Of. It. Otherwise, it's just taking up room in your mind and cupboards. Every time a trigger occurs, you have to battle the urge even if you and your mind both know it's there. Why subject yourself to that?

2. Get Rid of the Hidden Junk Food: Examine anything that is packaged or canned. Never believe cunning marketing claims such as "all-natural," "whole grains," or "100% healthy." These assertions are open to interpretation. Instead of making customers' health

better, the objective is to encourage them to buy the product.

3. Check the Ingredients List: Are the first few items whole grains? Even if you may be purchasing "gluten-free" treats, a deeper look at the ingredients may reveal that they are junk food.

4. Treat anything as a dessert if it has sugar as one of the first three components. This includes any of the "healthy" sugars, such as agave, honey, molasses, or molasses. All of it is sugar.

5. Verify how many grams of fiber are there. Although some goods increase the fiber content by adding cellulose (which isn't always a good thing), it is a sign of the product's integrity.

6. Keep an eye out for synthetic food dyes including red dye 40, yellow 5, and green. 3.

7. Does it include artificial sweeteners like xylitol, aspartame, or Splenda? Toss it.

8. Does it include trans fats, commonly known as partly hydrogenated oil,

shortening, or hydrogenated oil? Eliminate it.

Extra Credit: While you're cleaning out your pantry, write a list of the things you need to replace so you'll have it on hand when it's time to go shopping.

Creating a Supportive Environment

Your living and working environment is one of the basic elements of a weight reduction journey that is effective. Making healthy decisions may either be made simpler or more difficult by your environment. In this chapter, we'll look at how you might set up a setting that will promote and maintain your attempts to become in shape and live a better life.

- Clean Up Your Area

Living in a messy and disorderly environment might make you more stressed out and make it harder to concentrate on your health objectives. Start by cleaning up your house. Make a clean, relaxing atmosphere by getting rid of anything extra and organizing your possessions. A clutter-free environment may promote mental clarity and a more upbeat mindset, which makes it simpler to stick with your weight reduction program.

- Kitchen Renovation

About losing weight, your kitchen is the beating heart of your house. It's where you cook and keep your food, and it has a big impact on how you eat. Spend some time setting up your kitchen in a manner that advances your objectives:

1. Healthy Meals at Eye Level: Put wholesome items like fruits, vegetables, and whole grains in your refrigerator and pantry at eye level. This increases the likelihood that you'll choose these healthy selections.
2. Minimise Temptations: Remove or restrict the availability of processed meals and unhealthy, high-calorie snacks. You'll be

less prone to indulge if they're not easily accessible.

3. Portion Management Tools: Purchase measuring cups and a food scale to aid in precise portion management.

- Social Assistance

Having a supportive social network around you may make all the difference. Inform your loved ones about your desire to lose weight so they can support and inspire you. Think about joining an online forum or weight loss organization where you may meet others going through similar experiences. Having friends and family who can relate to your struggles and achievements may be quite beneficial.

- Meal Planning and Preparation

Meal planning and preparation is one of the greatest methods to create an atmosphere that supports weight reduction. Schedule time each week to make a grocery list, organize your meals, and prepare healthy snacks and supplies. When you have a variety of healthy alternatives at your disposal, you're less likely to make harmful decisions out of convenience or hunger.

- Exercice Area

If at all feasible, set aside a space in your house just for exercising. It doesn't have to be fancy; a yoga mat and some dumbbells in a corner of the room would do. Having a designated workout area may make it more comfortable to participate in regular physical activity and serve as a visible reminder of your dedication to health.

- Positive Affirmation and Visual Aids

Think about displaying inspirational sayings or positive affirmations throughout your house. Visual cues about your objectives might help you stay motivated and focused. Additionally, you might make a vision board with pictures of your ideal healthy lifestyle and the advantages of reaching your weight reduction objectives.

You'll position yourself for success on your weight reduction journey by fostering an atmosphere that supports healthy decisions and constructive behaviors. Keep in mind that even little adjustments to your environment may significantly boost your capacity to stay committed to your objectives and implement long-term lifestyle changes.

Chapter 2

Nutrition for Success

Whether you've been attempting to reduce weight for a few weeks or many years, it's simple to get discouraged if no progress is being made. The end effect is a never-ending struggle with the scale.

The fact is that dieting, eating less to reduce weight, and healthy nutrition are often confused. Unfortunately, most individuals are unaware of the significance of diet in terms of weight loss, which makes it more difficult to achieve health objectives.

Portion Control

Portion Control is a fantastic way to manage your healthy eating while also losing weight. This article defines portion management and provides a tonne of helpful advice on how to do it right to stay healthy.

One of the most effective nutrition tricks I've discovered for maintaining a healthy lifestyle, reducing weight, and reaching and maintaining my optimum weight is portion management. Knowing what your body requires can help you consume just what it requires. We overeat often, which causes weight gain, either because we feel obligated to finish everything on our plates or because restaurants provide pre-determined enormous servings.

Here comes portion management, which enables us to understand what is in our food and how much we should eat to achieve our objectives. However, a common misconception among those attempting to lose weight is that to do so, their food intake must be severely reduced. This isn't always the case.

The Power of Protein, Carbs, and Fats in a Balanced Diet

Fast food is often chosen because it is handy. Your body requires a complicated combination of nutrients, however, to feel and look your best. You also need enough fluids to be hydrated as well as a healthy serving of fiber in addition to the proper amounts of proteins, carbs, fats, vitamins, and minerals. Even the most conscientious eater may find it challenging to reach their daily nutritional goals.

Healthy foods and supplements that help you fulfill your daily requirements, together with the proper calorie balance to support weight loss, increase, or maintenance, are the foundation of balanced nutrition.

- **Protein**

A macronutrient called protein is essential for almost every cell in the body. You produce essential chemicals like hormones and enzymes as well as the building blocks of muscular tissue with the help of proteins. Protein is also quite effective in reducing hunger.

It's crucial to consume enough protein each day to replenish what your body has utilized as it builds, breaks down, and uses protein continually. We recommend getting up to 30% of your daily calories from lean protein sources including soy, chicken, fish, and eggs.

- **Carbohydrates**

Another macronutrient that your body wants to use as fuel is carbs, therefore it's critical to consume enough of these daily. Instead of the sweet, starchy carbohydrates found in soda, candy, and baked goods, we advise consuming around 40% of your calories from whole grains, beans, vegetables, and fruit.

- **Fat**

Additionally, your body needs trace quantities of healthy fats; but, hold off on going overboard just now; you probably already receive enough. The normal American diet has more total fat and saturated fat than humans need, as well as a deficiency in good fats like those found in fish, nuts, avocados, olive oil, and fish. Because fats are such a concentrated source of calories, the Herbalife Nutrition Philosophy advises consuming no more than 30% of your daily calories from fats.

You can manage both sides of the calorie equation when it comes to keeping your intake in check. By keeping track of the calories in the foods you consume, you can control how much goes in, and by being active, you can manage, at least in part, how many calories you burn each day. You can tip the scales whether you aim to lose, increase, or maintain weight.

Chapter 3

Meal Preparation and Planning

When attempting to reduce weight, meal planning and preparation may be an effective technique.

When carried out properly, it can assist you in achieving the calorie deficit necessary for weight loss while giving your body the nourishing foods it requires to function and maintain good health. Making your meals ahead of time can also speed up and streamline the preparation process.

When you initially begin meal planning, you could discover that you lose weight simply as a result of eating better and being more organized for mealtime. I've been meal planning on and off for the last five years and it's been a major component of self-care that has had some pretty wonderful advantages. As a consequence of being more organized with my meals, I've improved my general health and have even dropped some weight (around 25 pounds) while doing it!

Creating a 14-Day Meal Plan

Consider your week realistically before scheduling time for dinner preparation. The greatest healthy meal plans are those that fit with your schedule and general way of life, according to Stewart. Use pre-made meal plans like this one as a guide, and feel free to add in additional family favorites, repeat meals throughout the week, or use high-quality frozen items on days when you're very busy.

A free, customizable 14-day meal plan with a shopping list that includes breakfast, lunch, and supper.

	Breakfast	**Lunch**	**Dinner**	**Snacks**
Day 1	Muesil with Raspberries	White Bean and Vegetable Salad	Balsamic-Dijon Chicken with Wild Rice and Kale Salad	One Medium Apple
Day 2	Avocado Egg Toast	Turkey Meatballs with Spinach and	Squash and Red Lentil Curry	1 Medium Orange

		Feta Served On Seasoned Quinoa		
Day 3	Avocado, Prosciutto and Egg Sandwiches	Chicken Salad with Orzo and an Avocado-Lime Dressing	Lemon Couscous and Greek Seasoned Pork	Smoothies with Mango Beetroot, and Sweet Honey
Day 4	Toasted Bagels and	Mediterranean Orzo	Thai Green Seafood	Paleo Roasted Nuts

	Apple Breakfast Compote	Skillet	Curry	
Day 5	Sunny-Side Up Eggs, Avocado, Cheddar and Chives on Muesli	Power Kale Salad	Stir-fried Pork with Ginger and Delicata	Caprese Bruschetta
Day 6	Sweet Potato Waffles	Greek Spinach-Pasta Salad with Feta	Three Bean Enchiladas	1 cup of Banana Ice Cream

		Cheese and Beans		
Day 7	Honey-Lemon Cottage Cheese Pancakes	Black Bean Chipotle Tostadas	Greek Feta Hamburgers	Fudgy Black Bean Brownies
Day 8	Oats with Orange and Honey	Beef and Mushroom Ravioli Soup	Delicata Squash with Sausage	No-Bake Energy Bites
Day 9	Six-Grain Slow	Turkey-Quinoa	Roasted Salmon and	Low-Sugar Chocol

	Cooker Porridge	Salad	Farro Bowls	ate Chip Zucchini Muffins
Day 10	Tropical Fruit Smoothie Bowls	Grain and Veggie Bowls	Pork Chops, Apples, and Greens	Chocolate-Peanut Butter Granola Bar
Day 11	2 Egg Bites with Bacon and Spinach	Burrito Bowls	Chickpea Tikka Masala	Arugula Blt Pizza

Day 12	Apple and Almond Butter Panini	Burrito Bowls with Roasted Butternut Squash	I-Made-It-Myself Pizza	Confetti Peanut Butter Munchies
Day 13	Air-Fryer Breakfast Burritos	Turkey Meatball Grinder	Fish with Crispy Bread Crumbs, Spinach, and Onions	Chia Pudding
Day 14	Oatmeal with Peanut Butter,	Cheddar Toast and	Fruit Platter with Maple	Herbed Chicken, Orzo,

	Banana, and Bacon	Carrot-Apple Soup	Mascarpone Dip	and Zucchini

Shopping Advice

When making your weekly shopping list for weight reduction, give fruits, vegetables, and lean meats priority to aid with weight control. Continue reading for additional products to have on hand and ideas on how to utilize these goods to create wholesome meals, snacks, and treats.

Advice Before Shopping

Numerous benefits may be derived from preparation before food shopping. It might lessen the stress associated with planning your meals for the week. Additionally, you can guarantee that the menu selections accommodate everyone's dietary requirements or preferences.

When you make plans in advance, you'll also have the chance to save money. You'll have more time to examine any items that are on sale or seek coupons for things that you wish to buy. Additionally, shopping from what you already own saves you money by preventing the need to purchase additional food or materials.

Use a Wide Range of Ingredients

Pick a method for creating your shopping list. Prepare future shopping lists by considering the ingredients you'll need to prepare balanced meals and healthy snacks. Five ingredients may make up a well-rounded meal:

- Veggies: You may choose from fresh or frozen veggies.
- Lean protein: Keep in mind plant-based choices, such as frozen veggie burgers and lentils. Eggs are a fast and simple source of animal protein, as are canned salmon and tuna.
- Healthful fats: Extra virgin olive oil, olive tapenade, pesto made with olive oil,

avocado, nuts, nut butter, and tahini are a few healthy fats.

- Whole food carbohydrates: These include fresh or frozen fruit, starchy vegetables like potatoes, and whole grains like quinoa, oats, and brown rice. Pulses, a general word for beans, lentils, and chickpeas, provide both fiber-rich carbohydrates and protein.

- Natural seasonings: Seasonings may be made from fresh or dried herbs, spices, and other ingredients. They can also be made from healthy condiments like balsamic vinegar and stone-ground mustard.

- Dairy products may be a part of some of your meals, too. Choose soy milk, yogurts, and cheeses that are fortified or low-fat, fat-free, lactose-free, etc.

Make a menu-based shopping list.

Create a shopping list based on the ingredients you'll need for each meal and the store's divisions. You may use this technique to pack everything you need for dinner preparation when you return from your vacation. Then, all that is left to do is find the time to cook.

It might be helpful to pre-prepare so that all you have to do is plate and reheat your meal's components. According to one research conducted as part of a workplace weight control program, better weight reduction was linked to higher average meal planning frequency.

Decide on the Best Time to Shop

When you shop, it matters. You've undoubtedly heard that going grocery shopping on an empty stomach is not advised. You are more likely to make impulsive purchases while you are hungry than when you are full.

In addition to making you feel off-balance and less able to plan for your requirements, a rumbling stomach may make you feel distracted. Plan your trip for just after dinner so you won't feel hurried, and remember to carry your list.

Chapter 4

Exercise and Fitness

It is more successful to reduce weight by combining exercise and a nutritious diet than by relying alone on calorie restriction. A few illnesses' effects may be halted or even reversed by exercise. Exercise reduces cholesterol and blood pressure, which may help to stave against a heart attack.

Additionally, exercising reduces your chance of getting some malignancies, including colon and breast cancer. Exercise is also known to support feelings of confidence and well-being, perhaps reducing anxiety and depressive symptoms.

Exercise aids in weight reduction and weight maintenance. Exercise may boost metabolism, which is the amount of calories you burn each day. Lean body mass may be maintained and increased, which also contributes to a daily calorie burn rise.

The Role of Exercise in Weight Loss

As your activity levels rise, so does your body's need for fuel (calories), hence exercise is crucial to weight control. If your activity is following your ongoing eating strategy, it is very advantageous for keeping the weight off after it has been lost.

In addition to assisting you in achieving a healthy weight, it may help you avoid or even reverse the symptoms of certain illnesses, reduce blood pressure and cholesterol to lessen your chance of having a heart attack, build stronger bones (lowering your risk of fractures), and enhance your capacity for daily activities. The majority of people who lose weight by diet also gain it back within a year, which is the primary reason why physical activity and diet must be combined to help with weight control.

Knowing that research has been done on the link between exercise, weight, heart health, and lifespan is more crucial. According to the findings, exercise is "consistently associated with greater reductions in mortality risk" compared to weight loss. According to this research, inactive and obese men and women who exercise and improve their fitness have a reduced chance of dying prematurely by as much as 30%, even if they don't lose weight.

While you should strive for a calorie deficit, you should also keep in mind that you should consume all the nutrients your body requires and avoid using up too much of its energy since it needs some for daily activities and physical processes.

When exercising, you should still have a nutritious diet that is well-balanced so that your body gets all the nutrients it needs to operate. Exercise is essential for you to maintain movement in your body, gain strength and stamina, and control your weight and BMI.

Due to their additional weight, many obese individuals find it difficult to exercise. However, by gradually increasing physical activity, you may help to lose this extra weight, and as your fat cells go, your muscles should develop.

Your body needs strong muscles to maintain your bones and internal organs. Although muscle weighs more than fat, it is far better for your health. Exercise has been shown to support long-term weight maintenance, so you should schedule time for it each day, even if it means boarding the bus at a stop early or using the stairs at work rather than the elevator.

Any increase in physical activity is beneficial, and the less time you spend sitting down, the better for your health it is.

Creating a Workout Schedule

Exercise is a crucial part of the equation when it comes to reaching your weight reduction objectives. A good exercise routine not only aids in calorie burning but also enhances your general health and fitness. We'll walk you through the process of designing an exercise routine specifically for your weight reduction goals in this chapter.

- **Determine Your Fitness Level Currently**

It's critical to evaluate your present fitness level before creating your training routine. This will assist you in selecting the appropriate workout kinds and intensities. Think about the following elements:

1. Cardiovascular Fitness: How well are you able to maintain aerobic exercises like brisk walking, running, or cycling?
2. Strength and Endurance: How strong are you, and how many repetitions of various workouts are you able to complete?
3. Flexibility: To avoid injuries, it is important to evaluate your flexibility and mobility.

- **Set Specific Goals**

Establish your precise exercise and weight reduction objectives. Are you hoping to increase your general fitness, grow muscle, increase your stamina, or lose a certain amount of weight? Your training plan will be guided by setting specific, attainable goals, which will also keep you motivated.

- **Pick Your Exercises Carefully**

Your exercise routine should include a variety of aerobic, strength training, and flexibility activities for efficient weight reduction. Here are some alternatives to think about:

1. Cardiovascular Exercises: Exercises that help you burn calories and strengthen your heart including jogging, brisk walking, swimming, cycling, and dancing.
2. Strengthening Exercises: Utilising resistance training with weights, resistance bands, or your body weight can aid in gaining lean muscle mass. At rest, muscle burns more calories, which helps people lose weight.
3. Flexibility and Mobility Tasks: Stretching routines, yoga, and Pilates may increase

flexibility, lower the chance of injury, and improve general well-being.

- **Establish the Duration and Frequency of Your Workouts**

Try to complete at least 150 minutes of moderate-intensity aerobic exercise or 75 minutes of vigorous-intensity aerobic activity per week, as advised by health standards, to lose weight. Divide this into reasonable exercise periods. For instance, you may decide to work out five days a week for 30 minutes.

- **Establish a Weekly Workout Schedule**

Create a weekly fitness plan with a range of workouts. For instance:

1. Monday: cardio exercise (such as running or cycling)
2. Tuesday: strength training (such as a full-body workout)

3. Wednesday: rest or mild exercise (such as yoga or stretching).
4. Thursday: cardio exercise (such as swimming or brisk walking)
5. Friday: A strength training session (such as concentrating on various muscle groups)
6. On Saturday, engage in a cardio exercise (such as dancing or hiking).
7. On Sunday, relax or engage in light activities.

- **Development and Variety**

It's crucial to gradually push your body to notice benefits. As your fitness level rises, gradually increase the time, intricacy, or intensity of your exercises. Incorporate variation into your regimen as well to avoid monotony and plateaus.

- **Pay Attention to Your Body**

Finally, pay attention to your body. Stop working out immediately and get advice from a fitness expert or healthcare practitioner if you feel pain or discomfort. To avoid overuse injuries and guarantee long-term performance, rest and recuperation are crucial.

Staying Motivated

When attempting to lose weight, you could come into typical obstacles like sluggish progress or a weight loss plateau. But persevering will be rewarded in the long term.

Depending on why you want to lose weight, there are different ways to remain motivated. To ascertain if reducing weight is ideal for you and your specific health requirements, you should always visit a doctor before starting any weight reduction program.

Here are seven strategies for maintaining motivation when dieting:

- **Set SMART Goals**

Setting objectives is essential for weight reduction, according to Sydney Spiewak, a registered dietitian and nutritionist at Hartford, Connecticut's St. Francis Hospital and Medical

Centre. According to research, aiming for smaller objectives results in longer-lasting weight reduction than attempting to reduce weight without making any plans.

You may create realistic objectives and monitor your development by using the SMART approach. SMART is short for:

1. Specific: Avoid establishing excessively ambiguous objectives. Try using "I will increase my physical activity by 20 minutes each day" as an example rather than "I will exercise more."
2. Measurably: Establish objectives that are simple to measure, such as increasing your workout time or step count.
3. Achievable: Set specific, attainable objectives first, and then broaden from there. Start with a smaller manageable target, such as 20 minutes each day, if you'd want to exercise for up to an hour each day but are now unable to do so. As your endurance improves, progressively lengthen your workouts.

4. Relevant: Check that each objective is directly related to your overarching ambition to reduce weight. For instance, increased exercise is important for weight reduction, but restricting screen time is less important.

5. Time-related: Set a due date for each objective. As a result, you are held responsible and your progress is tracked. You may, for instance, make a plan to review your exercise habits once a month, assess your results, and then establish a new goal to increase your exercise the following month.

- **Locate a Friend**

According to Spiewak, having support from others makes losing weight simpler, particularly if you can locate a group of individuals who share your objectives. When you're having a hard time staying motivated, collaborating with friends or family who want to lose weight might help. You can keep each other accountable and encourage one other.

- **Engage in Mindfulness**

It entails paying attention to how your ideas, emotions, and physical experiences influence your actions.

According to Spiewak, mindfulness may be an effective strategy for creating healthy eating habits and lifestyle choices. This is so that we may slow down, pay attention to our feelings, and shut out distractions.

Consider how your meal tastes, and feels on your tongue, and what portion of it you like most, advises Spiewak. "This can help you be more mindful of the present moment by preventing you from overeating by preventing you from eating too soon.

- **Modify the Surroundings**

According to Spiewak, your environment must encourage you to make good decisions for weight reduction. You may do this by:

1. Fill your refrigerator with fresh produce, lean proteins, and dairy products.
2. Choosing restaurants that have a variety of nutritious foods
3. Laying out your workout attire before night.
4. Make a list before going food shopping. This will assist in reducing impulsive purchases and help you know precisely what to buy.

- **Make Exercise Enjoyable**

Exercise may be difficult. But according to Spiewak, you shouldn't push yourself to run if you don't like it.

The greatest method to exercise is to pick a regimen you can stay with and enjoy:

You may discover various dance exercises online, like Zumba, if you love dancing. Take walks while increasing your speed and distance if you prefer exercising outside. Don't be hesitant to experiment with various routines, such as kickboxing or yoga, until you discover one you prefer.

- **Consider Maintaining a Food Journal**

Making a food journal holds you responsible and identifies areas for improvement. You may identify patterns or particular triggers that can lead you to stray from your path by keeping a food journal.

- **Be Kind to Yourself**

According to Spiewak, losing weight is challenging and often not a linear process. It's typical to encounter plateaus or even sporadic weight increases.

"Life is not perfect, your weight loss journey will contain setbacks, but it will also contain great triumphs," Spiewak asserts. It is crucial to constantly remind yourself that you are a human being.

It's important to be kind to oneself after a failure. Your commitment to your long-term objectives should take precedence over trying to achieve daily excellence in the face of a sickness or a difficult workday.

"An all-or-nothing mindset is detrimental to achieving your goals," Spiewak claims. Your diet will sometimes fall short of perfection. You could not have had time to prepare your meals or you might want a piece of cake since it's your birthday. Permit yourself to do so, and then return to your plan for the next meal or the following day.

Chapter 5

Motivation and Attitude

It takes more than simply making physical adjustments to lose weight; you also need to have the correct attitude and maintain motivation throughout the process. This chapter will discuss the critical role that motivation and attitude play in effective weight reduction and provide you with tips on how to have a good frame of mind.

- **Identify Your Motives**

Spend some time thinking about why you want to lose weight before starting your weight-loss journey. Your "why" acts as your motivation and helps keep you focused when difficulties arise. Knowing your why is crucial, whether it's to improve your health, increase your confidence, set a good example for your loved ones, or just feel better in your body.

- **Establish Realistic Goals**

While having lofty objectives is important, they should also be attainable and reasonable. Setting impossible objectives may cause disappointment and demotivation. Divide your ultimate objective into smaller, easier-to-achieve stages. Celebrate your accomplishments along the road to maintain your drive.

- **Visualize Success**

An effective technique for keeping motivation high is visualization. Every day, set aside some time to visualize your accomplishment. Imagine reaching your ideal weight and feeling confident and in good health. Your dedication may be strengthened and your objectives might seem more accessible with the assistance of visualization.

- **Be Optimistic**

Positivity can make all the difference. Think about the advantages of your travel rather than what you can't have or are giving up. Every positive decision you make, no matter how tiny, should be celebrated. Remind yourself that you are moving in the direction of a better, happier you.

- **Recover from Failures**

Failures are a common occurrence in any weight reduction program. Consider their chances to learn and develop as opposed to failures. Determine what went wrong and take the opportunity to change your strategy and make better decisions going ahead.

- **Surround Yourself with Supportive People**

Having a strong support system around you may make all the difference. Share your objectives with loved ones so they can support and understand you. Consider signing up for a weight reduction support group or consulting a mentor or coach who can provide direction and responsibility.

- **Exercise Self-Compassion**

Throughout your journey, be sensitive and nice to yourself. There may be times of annoyance and self-doubt while trying to lose weight. You should treat yourself with the same compassion and understanding that you would provide to a friend going through a similar situation.

- **Stay Current**

Knowing something is a great motivation. Keep learning more about healthy eating, exercise, and life. Knowing the science underlying weight reduction and the advantages of a healthy lifestyle will help you stay more committed to your objectives.

- **Rejoice in Your Successes**

As you attain your milestones, stop to recognize your success. Celebrations don't have to revolve around food; they may include incentives like investing in new exercise equipment, spoiling yourself with a day at the spa, or engaging in a passion project unrelated to food that you love.

- **Discover Joy in the Journey**

Finally, keep in mind that enjoying the process is just as important as accomplishing your goal when it comes to losing weight. Discovering new, nutritious foods, finding physical activities you like, and seeing the good changes in your body and mind may all be enjoyable.

Overcoming Obstacle

Losing weight may be stressful and difficult, particularly if you run across roadblocks that make it more difficult or halt your progress. Fortunately, you may overcome these challenges and accomplish your weight-loss objectives by adopting the appropriate mentality and tactics. Keep in mind that you are more than a weight on a scale. Being healthy and attaining your objectives depends greatly on how confident you are in your abilities.

Here are some strategies for doing so:

- **Time Restrictions**

Lack of time is a major obstacle while attempting to reduce weight. Finding time to work out, prepare wholesome meals, and take care of yourself may be challenging when you have to juggle your job, family obligations, and other commitments. However, it's crucial to put your health first.

Try the following advice:

1. Make a schedule for your exercises and food preparation time. You may ensure that you carve out time only for these hobbies in this manner.
2. Get assistance from your loved ones or friends. They may assist you by splitting the effort, such as doing the cooking and cleaning, leaving you with more free time.

- **Eat Out of Emotion**

Another frequent barrier that might make it difficult to lose weight is emotional eating. When feeling down or worried, many individuals resort to food as a coping technique, which may result in overeating and weight gain.

To stop emotional eating, use these suggestions:

1. Recognize the triggers for your need to eat even when you're not hungry. Is it a specific feeling or circumstance? Knowing your triggers can help you develop healthy methods to handle them.

2. If you feel like eating but aren't genuinely hungry, take a moment. Take 10 full breaths while closing your eyes. How can you care for yourself without utilizing food or drink? Ask yourself what emotion you are experiencing. Try practicing stress-relieving exercises like yoga, meditation, or journal writing.

3. Talking to a therapist or joining a support group might also be beneficial. They can help you overcome your emotional eating patterns by offering advice and compassion.

- **Plateau**

Hitting a plateau, which may last weeks or even months, is another item that might hinder weight loss. Even after making progress at first, it might be demoralizing to see no changes in your weight or physical appearance. But reaching a plateau is common throughout the weight-loss process, so it's crucial to be patient and consistent.

Here are some ideas for breaking through a plateau:

1. Consider switching up your fitness regimen. It's wise to switch things up since your body could have become used to the same activities. You may experiment with new things or step up the intensity of your routines.
2. Make calorie intake adjustments. Your body may sometimes need a little prodding to go beyond a plateau. You may try eating fewer calories or include more nutrient-dense foods in your diet.

3. Replace one normal meal with a meal replacement product, such as a frozen meal, nutrition bar, or meal replacement shake, as a simple nutrition plan. Do this every day for 30 days, choose one with less than 300 calories. This may help you control your caloric consumption while still ensuring that you get the right nourishment.

- **Social Constraints**

It may be challenging to reduce weight due to social influences. Peers or friends may sometimes put pressure on you to engage in unhealthy behaviors or attend gatherings with a lot of food and alcohol. In certain circumstances, maintaining your weight-loss objectives might be challenging. But keep in mind that you are the one who makes the decisions, and your health comes first.

The following advice can help you deal with societal pressure:

1. Take your wholesome food to social gatherings
2. Suggest engaging in non-food-related activities with your pals so that you'll have something nourishing to eat and won't feel as tempted to consume unhealthy foods. You may play a sport, go on a stroll, or have a game night. In this manner, you may still spend time together without making food the main topic.
3. Keep in mind that declining an invitation is acceptable. If peer pressure conflicts with your objectives, you don't have to give in. Keep your choices strong and give your health priority.

- **Remain Steadfast**

Although losing weight might be challenging, you can overcome these difficulties and accomplish your objectives by maintaining a positive outlook and using effective tactics. Always remember that your health should come first and how crucial it is to look after yourself. If you are aware of the factors that make it difficult for you to remain on track, strive to avoid them. And if you want assistance, don't be hesitant to ask for it. You can achieve your objectives and have a healthy life if you are persistent and laser-focused.

Having a Positive Attitude

Both mental and physical effort are required to lose weight. It requires commitment, dedication, and a significant amount of mental effort to get out of bed every morning and adhere to your food and exercise objectives. Even while it might be taxing on your body to push through a workout, it's seldom your arms or legs that start to urge you to stop. When it comes to giving up on your goal of losing weight, that inner voice is often to blame.

One of the most important weapons you can use to lose weight is an optimistic outlook. You may recall the proverb you heard as a youngster that goes, "Sticks and stones may break my bones, but words shall never harm me." If only that were accurate! When it comes to reducing weight, negativity may reduce your preparedness and drive to improve your health. Negative comments can have a significant negative influence on your willingness to achieve.

It takes time to cultivate a powerful, optimistic mentality. It is difficult to transition to a positive frame of mind after years of hating yourself and concentrating only on the flaws in your physical appearance. From Los Angeles to Bakersfield, there will be individuals and locations that will trigger unpleasant memories and undermine your optimistic outlook. A little setback is OK. Take those possibilities for growth, and then do everything you can to advance.

Being optimistic is more crucial than ever while undergoing a medical weight reduction program. Here are some tips to help you maintain a positive outlook when trying to lose weight:

1. Be more grateful for the little things in life that make you happy. A nice drink of cold

water on a hot day or the way a family member makes you giggle might be examples of this.

2. Increase the things you like doing. Don't be afraid to indulge in your passions. Go ahead and start a new pastime, take up a hobby, or just read a book.

3. Encourage yourself by preparing to learn something new each day. Every day presents a new learning opportunity. Take the time to learn something new; it could alter your perspective on the world and provide you with something to ponder.

Being consistently optimistic might take some practice, but in the meantime, you can try to maintain a happy attitude and fend off any pessimistic ideas that can slow down your weight reduction efforts. During your medical weight reduction program, push yourself to be healthy and surround yourself with encouraging people. Don't underestimate this sort of healthy mentality since it's just as important to your medical weight reduction program as making dietary and activity improvements.

Chapter 6

Tracking Progress

It's crucial to monitor your weight reduction progress for several reasons. You can make the required modifications and get insightful information about your progress thanks to it. We'll look at some efficient strategies to monitor your progress in this section.

- **Weighing Yourself**

One of the most popular ways to keep tabs on your weight reduction progress is to weigh yourself often. However, it's crucial to approach it properly:

1. The frequency: Weighing oneself at the same time each day under comparable circumstances, for as just after using the loo in the morning, is recommended. Many individuals choose to weigh themselves once every week to monitor trends rather than daily changes.

2. Pay attention to trends: Recognise that everyday variations in weight are common and may be impacted by things like hydration, food, and exercise. Instead of focusing on the specific daily data, consider the overall trend.

- **Measurements of the Body**

You may get a more complete picture of your development by taking measurements of several body sections, such as your waist, hips, chest, arms, and thighs. You may see changes in measures as you lose fat and build muscle, even if the scale doesn't reflect any appreciable improvements.

- **Progress Pictures**

Using before-and-after pictures to illustrate your shift may be quite effective. Taking pictures:

1. Use consistent lighting: Make sure the lighting is the same in both images to properly compare changes.

2. Wear the same clothing: To remove clothing-related factors, wear the same clothes in each photograph.

3. Take pictures from several perspectives: Record front, side, and rear shots to get a full picture of your development.

- **Maintaining a Journal**

By keeping a weight loss notebook, you may track other parts of your journey outside just your weight, like:

1. Keep track of your meals, snacks, and portion sizes. You may recognize your eating habits and make changes as a result.

2. Record your workouts, noting their length, level of difficulty, and kind of activity.

3. Emotions and triggers: Take note of your emotional state and any circumstances that may affect your eating habits.

- **Fitness Evaluations**

You may track advancements in your strength, endurance, flexibility, and cardiovascular fitness with regular fitness examinations. To monitor your development over time, you might engage with a fitness expert or take standardized fitness tests.

- **Health Indicators**

Monitoring your health indicators, such as blood pressure, cholesterol, and blood sugar levels, may provide you with important information about how you are doing overall. These metrics may be effective success indicators if they improve.

- **Tracking Applications and Tools**

There are several tools and applications available that may be used to quickly monitor your progress. These applications often let you log your eating habits, exercise routines, and measurements while also showing you visual representations of your development.

- **Consulting Experts**

To analyze your progress objectively, think about speaking with a medical expert or certified nutritionist. They may provide advice on monitoring techniques and assist you in interpreting your data in light of your unique health and objectives.

- **Setting Goals and Milestones**

Set up clear checkpoints along the way to your weight reduction. These could have to do with your weight, your level of exercise, or other facets of your health. Celebrating these achievements might inspire you and make you feel accomplished.

Using Technology to Stay on Track

Everybody who is attempting to reduce weight should have certain tools to assist them in staying on track. Being overweight is not exactly simple. To make significant changes in your lifestyle, such as changing your food and engaging in a lot of physical exercise, you need to be completely committed and motivated.

You can use technology to simplify your weight reduction journey a little bit. You may purchase some fitness tools to aid you in your weight reduction quest, ranging from monitoring your caloric intake to selecting the best weighing scale. You've come to the correct place if you've been seeking devices to help you lose weight. We've put together a list of some of the top technologies you may utilize to aid with weight loss.

Depending on your demands, choose the top technology for weight reduction.

Here are some of the top tools you need to get to lose those excess pounds:

This section will look at how you can successfully use technology to help your weight reduction goals.

- **Apps for food and diet**

There are several diet and nutrition applications available that may help you keep track of your calorie consumption, measure your food intake, and make educated dietary decisions. Chronometer, Lose It!, and MyFitnessPal are a few well-liked choices. These programs can determine your daily caloric requirements depending on your objectives and often have large food databases.

- **Apps for physical activity and fitness**

You can plan, monitor, and vary your exercises with the aid of fitness apps. Numerous of these applications include reminders, progress monitoring, and guided exercise regimens to help you stay responsible. For recording outdoor activities like running and cycling, examples include Strava, Fitbod, and Nike Training Club.

- **Wearable fitness devices**

Smartwatches and other fitness wearables, like fitness trackers, may provide you with real-time information on your activity levels, heart rate, sleep habits, and other things. You can track your progress and establish objectives since they connect with the appropriate smartphone applications. Popular alternatives include Fitbit, Apple Watch, and Garmin.

- **Apps for meal planning and recipe searching**

The task of drafting nutrient-dense, balanced meal plans may be made easier by meal planning applications. Some applications even create shopping lists depending on the recipes you've chosen. Yummly, and Plan to Eat are a few examples.

- **Social media and online communities**

Social media platforms and online weight loss forums may be a great source of support and accountability. You may update others on your progress, connect with those on a similar path to you, and draw inspiration and motivation from other people's experiences.

- **Mindfulness and meditation apps**

It's crucial to control stress and emotional eating if you want to lose weight. You may build relaxation strategies and mindfulness practices to enhance your mental and emotional well-being by using mindfulness and meditation applications like Headspace and Calm.

- **Virtual coaches and personal trainers**

Consider working with virtual personal trainers or coaches if you desire tailored advice. Numerous experts provide online coaching services, creating individualized training and diet programs based on your unique objectives.

- **Online meal delivery and ordering services**

Investigate online food delivery businesses that provide wholesome meal alternatives to make eating healthy more easy. The delivery of goods and recipes to your home by companies like HelloFresh, Blue Apron, and Purple Carrot makes dinner preparation simpler and more pleasant.

- **Health-tracking applications**

You may monitor important health metrics like blood pressure, blood sugar, and cholesterol levels with health monitoring applications. They may aid in tracking your development and assisting you and your healthcare practitioner in making wise choices about your health.

- **Smart scales and body composition monitors**

Beyond only weight, smart scales and body composition analyzers provide thorough insights into your body's makeup. They often measure things like muscle mass and body fat percentage. Some sync with mobile applications to monitor changes over time.

Chapter 7

Lifestyle Modifications

Making permanent lifestyle adjustments is often necessary to lose weight and keep it off in addition to diets and exercise. We'll examine important lifestyle changes that may support effective weight reduction and long-term weight control in this section.

- **Balanced Nutrition**

A balanced diet is essential for losing weight. Make the dietary adjustments listed below:

1. Portion Control: Watch your portions to prevent overeating. Use smaller dishes, plates, and utensils to help you manage your portions.
2. Emphasize Healthy Foods: Base your meals on healthy grains, lean meats, fruits, and vegetables. These meals provide the necessary nutrients and are more satisfying.

3. Reduce the amount of processed and highly refined foods you consume. These foods are often heavy in added sugars, bad fats, and empty calories.
4. Drink plenty of water all day long. Sometimes, hunger and thirst are confused.

- **Consistent Physical Activity**

Regular physical exercise must be a part of your everyday routine if you want to lose weight:

1. Set Realistic Goals: Begin with workable fitness objectives and progressively raise the length and intensity of your exercises.
2. Select Interest You Have : No matter whether you like dancing, walking, cycling, dancing, or playing a sport, choose physical activities you love. Consistent activity will be simpler to maintain as a result.
3. Strengthening Exercise: To gain muscle, which helps accelerate your metabolism, use strength training workouts in your daily regimen.

4. Consistency is essential: Strive for consistency in your exercise regimen, aiming for at least 150 minutes per week of aerobic activity at a moderate level.

- **Mindful Eating Practices**

You can better regulate your food intake and your connection with food by adopting mindful eating practices:

1. Eat Slowly: Enjoy every mouthful and pay attention to your body's signals of hunger and fullness.
2. Avoid Distractions: To minimize mindless overeating, limit distractions while eating, such as television, cellphones, or laptops.
3. Practice Portion Awareness: To assist in managing portion sizes, use smaller plates and utensils. You can also think about pre-portioning snacks.

- **Adequate Sleep**

The importance of getting enough sleep for general health and weight reduction

1. Make Sleep a Priority: Aim for 7-9 hours of restful sleep each night. Hormones that control appetite may be disturbed by sleep deprivation, which can result in increased desires and weight gain.

2. Establish a routine by Setting a consistent bedtime and wake-up time each day to establish a regular sleep routine.

- **Stress Management**

Ongoing stress might cause emotional eating and weight gain.

1. Identify Stressors: Recognise the stressors in your life and identify constructive coping mechanisms, including deep breathing exercises, hobbies, or meditation.

2. Seek Support: If stress plays a big part in your life, think about getting help from a therapist or counselor.

- **Social Accountability and Support**

Make use of your social network to aid your weight reduction efforts:

1. Share Your Goals: Let friends and family know what your objectives are so they can support you and show compassion.
2. Find an Accountability Partner: Take into account collaborating with a friend or relative who has like objectives.

- **Long-Term Perspective**

To lose weight successfully, keep in mind that you must adjust your lifestyle and habits to maintain the weight reduction you achieve. Change the direction of your attention to a long-term, sustainable strategy for health and wellbeing.

- **Professional Directions**

Think about getting advice from a trained dietician or healthcare provider. They may provide you with individualized guidance, track your development, and assist you in making wise choices about your weight reduction endeavor.

Healthy Habits for Long-Term Success

Starting a weight reduction journey may be scary, but establishing the proper behaviors to support long-term success is just half the fight. Many of us are attracted to adopting fad diets because we want to see results as soon as possible. These often work only momentarily and are seldom long-lasting, and many individuals eventually put on even more weight as a result.

- **Keep a Food Journal**

Keeping a food diary might be unexpected since many of us are unaware of what we consume daily. We can discover that we consume a lot more harmful meals than we first believed. Because of this, keeping track of your dietary intake is crucial while attempting to alter and better understand your eating patterns.

- **Reduce Dining Out**

Although fast food and takeaway are typically filled with toxic substances that aren't good for our bodies, they may be handy. Furthermore, several studies have shown that eating fast food contributes to weight growth.

Putting a limit on how often you dine out may help you lose weight. Unlike eating out, when you can't be sure exactly what is in your food when you cook your meals at home, you have far more control over the ingredients and quantities that you use.

- **Create a Support Network**

Trying to lose weight on your own might be difficult. Sharing your success with friends, family, or even a weight reduction club may assist with accountability and support.

This is supported by research, which has shown that seeing others' success in weight reduction programs may inspire and drive people, increasing their likelihood of losing weight. So, be sure to motivate yourself along the road and share your adventure with a buddy or a group.

- **Obtain Enough Sleep**

When establishing healthy weight reduction habits, sleep must always come first. A restful night's sleep controls metabolism and hunger hormones, preventing overeating.

An adult requires, on average, 7-9 hours of sleep per night. If you don't get enough, attempt to establish a regular sleep schedule that suits you. Whatever you need to do to have a restful night's sleep, such as turning off your phone, listening to an audiobook, or taking a soothing bath.

- **Reduce Stress Levels**

Stress may sabotage your efforts to lose weight by making you want comfort foods and causing your body to accumulate fat as a reaction to the stress. Additionally, it may alter metabolism and lead to emotional eating.

Luckily, there are methods for reducing excessive levels of stress. You may experiment with attentive activities like yoga or meditation. Additionally, regular exercise supports weight reduction while enhancing mood and acting as a natural stress reliever.

Never undervalue the impact of a hearty laugh or time spent with loved ones. Remember that maintaining mental health is just as important for weight reduction as food and exercise.

- **Making a Meal Plan in Advance**

Planning and preparing meals in advance is a simple habit you can form. A game-changer, meal preparation ensures balanced, portion-controlled meals and prevents impulsive, unhealthy food choices.

Start by creating a weekly meal with an emphasis on wholesome, satisfying foods. Spend a few hours a week cooking and portioning, after that. Purchase high-quality storage containers to facilitate quick grab-and-go meals. Making lasting, straightforward meals that support your nutritional objectives is the key.

- **Drink Plenty of Water**

You must drink more water, as you are probably well aware. Water is an excellent source of nutrients for our organs, energy, and hunger satiation. It may also help us lose weight. Even now and again, some mistake hunger signs for thirst cues.

Carrying a reusable water bottle around might help you drink more water by encouraging frequent sips. Do you find water boring? For more flavor, add fruits, herbs, or a dash of juice to your water. Additionally, try to remember to sip a glass of water before each meal by setting reminders on your phone.

- **Eat at Regular Meal Times**

Late-night cravings may be quite strong and often interfere with weight reduction efforts and lead to overeating. Additionally, the body naturally slows down its metabolism at night, which results in less effective calorie burning.

Attempt to eat consistently throughout the day. Breakfast needs to be had within an hour after waking up, and supper ought to be consumed several hours before bed. Studies suggest that meals that begin around 5 p.m. may be advantageous. To achieve maximum metabolic performance, eating habits should be coordinated with your body's circadian cycle.

- **Exercise Each Day**

Undoubtedly, physical exercise is very important for effective, long-lasting weight reduction. Since many of us lead sedentary lives, it's crucial to make sure we're receiving the necessary exercise.

The American Department of Health and Human Services advises individuals to engage in 150 minutes of vigorous physical exercise per week. Anyone can fit in extra exercise throughout the day, regardless of their schedule or access to a gym. Include at-home exercises in your routine or try HIIT as a fast and efficient approach to begin moving and boost your heart rate.

- **Discover Balanced Diets**

A balanced diet may be among the most crucial weight reduction practices. Eating nutritious, nutrient-dense meals may promote satiety, a balanced relationship with food, and improved bodily performance.

Lean meats, entire grains, an abundance of fruits and vegetables, and healthy fats make up a balanced diet. The key is moderation and variety. Limiting processed meals and sugary snacks is also a good idea since they often contain a lot of empty calories.

- **Put Portion Control First**

A lot of the time, how much you eat rather than what you consume is the issue. To avoid overeating, even for nutritious meals, portion management is essential for weight reduction.

Use smaller plates to deceive your brain into thinking you can eat less to conquer it. Put veggies on half of your plate, lean protein on the other half, and whole grains on the last quarter. Lastly, to increase enjoyment and recognize fullness indicators, savor each mouthful while eating attentively.

- **Register Your Body's Hunger Cues**

Are you really hungry, or are you simply feeling emotional, irritated, bored, or tired? Sometimes, what we interpret as a hunger indication is something quite different. The body's natural signs to eat, such as a rumbling stomach or low energy, are known as hunger cues. Contrarily, emotional eating is motivated by stress, boredom, or grief.

Understanding the difference between actual and fictitious hunger is essential for long-term weight reduction. Unlike physical hunger, which grows gradually, emotional hunger generally hits all at once.

- **Spend Time in the Sun**

In addition to improving our mood and keeping us healthy, vitamin D also aids in weight loss by controlling hunger and fat accumulation. According to a 2018 research, participants' BMI considerably decreased after taking a vitamin D supplement for six weeks.

So how can you increase your vitamin D intake even when you spend most of the day indoors? Start by opening the blinds and taking little breaks outside. Additionally, the sunlight and fresh air help to reduce tension.

- **Always Eat a Filling Breakfast**

Keep in mind that breakfast is the most crucial meal of the day and that it must include the correct foods.

To aid with hunger levels and satiety, protein is important to eat first thing in the morning. If bread or cereal is your usual morning fare, think about including a protein-rich dish to balance your meal.

Greek yogurt with fruit and nuts, a protein drink with berries, or an omelet with your preferred vegetables are a few examples.

Sleep, Stress, and Weight Loss

The relationships between sleep, stress, and weight reduction are complex and significant. Understanding these connections may guide your decision-making and assist your weight reduction objectives.

- **The Importance of Sleep for Weight Loss**

An essential element of healthy weight reduction is getting enough sleep. The impact of sleep on metabolism and weight is as follows:

1. Hormone Balance: Hormones that influence hunger and appetite are regulated by sleep. Lack of sleep causes your body to create more of the hunger hormone ghrelin and less of the hormone

leptin, which increases cravings and overeating.

2. Control of Blood Sugar: Lack of sleep may impair insulin sensitivity, raising blood sugar levels and causing more fat to be stored.

3. Energy Levels You may feel worn out and less inspired to exercise if you get poor-quality sleep.

4. Emotional Eating: Lack of sleep may cause emotional eating because your body searches for immediate energy solutions, often in the form of sweet or high-calorie meals.

5. Snacks to Enjoy Late at Night: Staying up late increases the likelihood of late-night eating, which often entails poor options.

- **Recommendations for Better Sleep**

Your attempts to lose weight may be favorably impacted by getting better sleep:

Establishing a sleep schedule can help your body's internal clock to run smoothly. Do this every day, including on weekends, by going to bed and waking up at the same time.

1. Create an Environment That Is Sleep-Friendly: Ensure that your bedroom is quiet, cool, and dark. Purchase a comfortable mattress and pillows.
2. Limit your screen time by avoiding using screens (phones, laptops, and TVs) at least an hour before going to bed because the blue light they generate may disrupt the synthesis of melatonin, a hormone that controls sleep.
3. Limit Alcohol and Caffeine: Reduce coffee and alcohol intake in the hours before bed since they might interfere with sleep cycles.
4. Regular Exercise: Getting regular exercise will help you sleep better. But stay away from strenuous exertion just before night.

- **The Effect of Stress on Losing Weight**

Weight reduction may be significantly hampered by persistent stress. How stress impacts your weight is as follows:

1. Emotional Eating: Emotional eating is a common response to stress to deal with unpleasant feelings.
2. Hormonal Alterations: Cortisol, a stress hormone, may rise as a result of prolonged stress. Increased cortisol levels may encourage the accumulation of fat, especially around the abdomen.
3. Routine Disrupted: Your usual food and exercise schedules may be disrupted by stress, making it difficult to stick to healthy patterns.

- **Stress Management for Weight Loss**

Developing excellent stress management skills may help you lose weight:

1. Use these stress-reduction strategies: Reduce stress levels by using relaxation

methods like yoga, deep breathing exercises, or meditation.

2. Practice: Regular exercise may be a great way to reduce stress. Endorphins are released, which improve mood and lessen stress.

3. Time Management: Plan your day to minimize pressures and prevent scheduling overload.

4. Seek Assistance: If you have chronic stress, don't be afraid to ask friends, family, or a professional for help.

5. Prioritise Self-Care: Schedule frequent breaks and indulge in relaxing activities to make self-care a priority.

Social Support and Accountability

Physically losing weight is difficult, but it's also stressful emotionally. The emotion of weight loss may be a great burden, whether it's adapting to a new lifestyle, starting new habits, or coping with the difficulties of plateaus.

Having someone to depend on when the going gets rough might be one of the most important advantages of a social network. You can get through challenging times by drawing on the knowledge and experiences of others. Allow people to assist you in your weight loss efforts by drawing on their prior knowledge and achievements.

You Have Support in Real Life

The daily assistance you need to sustain success comes from friends and family, which is one of the most tangible types of support. Others may assist you in a variety of ways, like by providing transportation to the gym, watching the kids while you go for a run, or assisting you in preparing nutritious meals for yourself.

Recognize the little ways your loved ones can support you along the path. They can ensure that there are few obstacles on your path to success.

You Have People to Keep You Accountable

The capacity to retain responsibility is maybe the most important advantage of a social support network for your weight reduction quest. It's simple to maintain a diet and an exercise plan for a few weeks, but individuals often give up before reaching their weight-loss goal. A strong social network can help you stay accountable and motivated to succeed.

This might take the shape of people working out with you to keep you motivated or just saying encouraging things to keep going. It's important to be determined, and it's simpler to go on when you have support from others.

You Must Continually Look for Help

Always be aware of your standards and the effort needed to achieve your objectives. Consult a physician who specializes in weight reduction for assistance in creating a healthy and practical weight loss program. (Trying to do it alone may result in a lot of failures and needless stress.)

Conclusion: Your Ongoing Weight Loss Journey

Your path to losing weight is a continuous, dynamic process that requires commitment, tenacity, and self-care. It's crucial to understand that your dedication to health and well-being doesn't cease as you finish this book. Instead, it ushers in a lifetime of progress toward a better, happier self.

Here are some salient conclusions and closing ideas to keep in mind as you continue your weight reduction journey:

- Being Consistent Throughout: Consistency is necessary for healthy living and sustainable weight loss. Continue to make healthy eating a priority and include regular exercise in your daily routine.
- Mindful Decisions: Maintain awareness of your dietary preferences, portion amounts, and eating routines. Overindulgence may

be avoided through mindful eating, which promotes a better connection with food.

- Maintain an active lifestyle by partaking in workouts and pursuits you find enjoyable. Regular physical exercise not only supports weight control but also improves general health.
- Prioritise your well-being. Take good care of your emotional and mental well-being. Your path must include stress reduction, enough sleep, and relaxation practices.
- Non-Scale Successes: Celebrate achievements outside weight loss, such as increased vitality, self-assurance, and general health. The results on the scale are not more significant than these accomplishments.
- Establish New Objectives: Set new objectives when you attain your original weight reduction targets to maintain your desire and advance.
- Maintain Your Knowledge: Maintain your knowledge of diet, exercise, and health.

You can make wise decisions when you are well-informed.

- Seek Assistance: Lean on your network of friends, family, and/or professionals as support. Their support and advice may be really helpful.

- Embrace Change: Recognise that life is a perpetual state of change. Accept it and learn to adjust as you go along to new situations and difficulties.

- Self-Compassion: Be nice to yourself, particularly when you have plateaus or setbacks. Self-compassion enables you to recover and maintain your commitment.

Workout Plans

Creating a 14-day weight loss work plan requires a more focused and intensive approach. An example schedule for a 14-day weight reduction program is shown below:

By following a well-organized schedule for the next 14 days, the goal is to jump-start your weight reduction.

Calendar: 14 days

Day 1-2: Setting the Scene

Objective: For the forthcoming 14-day program, get yourself emotionally and physically ready.

Tasks:

- ☐ Take "before" pictures to measure development.
- ☐ Eliminate any unhealthy food from your kitchen.
- ☐ Buy supplies for dinner preparation and groceries.

☐ For the next 14 days, set precise weight reduction objectives.

Moves:

☐ Determine a calorie deficit for weight reduction by calculating your daily caloric requirements.
☐ Design a 14-day menu with an emphasis on a balanced diet.
☐ Plan daily workouts for the next two weeks.

Day 3–7: Nutrition and Diet Focus

Goal: Create wholesome eating routines that support weight reduction.

Tasks:

☐ Strictly adhere to the earlier-made food plan.
☐ Carefully monitor your dietary intake with a nutrition app or notebook.
☐ Pay attention to portion management and refrain from between-meal snacking.

☐ Try out fresh, healthful dishes to keep mealtime interesting.

Moves:

☐ Eat a diet high in fruits, vegetables, whole grains, and lean proteins.
☐ Drink a lot of water throughout the day to stay hydrated.
☐ Cut sugar and processed food out of your diet.
☐ Permit yourself one tiny indulgence on a set day to avoid feeling deprived.

Day 8-Day 11: Intensive Exercise

Goals: Incorporate rigorous exercise to increase metabolism and calorie burn.

Tasks:

☐ Stick to the earlier-set training regimen.
☐ Increase your workout's length and intensity.
☐ Combine workouts for your strength, flexibility, and cardiovascular system.

☐ Continue to follow your workout regimen consistently.

Moves:

☐ Aim for 60 minutes or more of moderate to vigorous activity each day.
☐ Perform strength training activities three to four times each week to maintain lean muscle mass.
☐ Pick exercises that are challenging for you to keep your workouts interesting.

Day 12-Day 14: Monitoring and Wrap-Up

Goal: Evaluate your progress, make any required modifications, and end the 14-day program.

Tasks:

☐ Examine your progress in losing weight and acknowledge accomplishments.
☐ Take into account any difficulties or roadblocks you experienced.

- ☐ Make necessary adjustments to your diet and exercise schedule.
- ☐ Make plans for maintenance and continuation beyond the 14 days.

Moves:

- ☐ Keep tabs on your dietary consumption and activity.
- ☐ If necessary, seek expert advice (such as a meeting with a licensed dietician).
- ☐ Establish new, long-term objectives to keep your weight reduction going beyond the first 14 days.
- ☐ Keep yourself motivated, engaged, and dedicated to the 14-day program by engaging in ongoing support and self-care throughout the program.

Tasks:

- ☐ Rely on your support network for accountability and motivation.
- ☐ Use stress-reduction strategies like deep breathing and meditation.

- [ ] Prioritize getting enough rest and sleep for recuperation.
- [ ] Keep track of your development and non-scale successes.

Moves:

- [ ] Maintain discipline and follow the diet plan and exercise schedule.
- [ ] Remind yourself often of your objectives and motivations for starting the 14-day program.
- [ ] Celebrate little accomplishments to keep inspired.
- [ ] Keep in mind that this 14-day program is just a kickstart, and sustained success requires a more long-term strategy.

This 14-day work schedule is created to provide a methodical and targeted strategy for losing weight. To be sure it's secure and appropriate for your particular circumstances, please speak with a medical expert or certified nutritionist before beginning any aggressive short-term weight reduction program.

Recipes Plan and Ideas

Here are some meals and meal suggestions that are both nutritious and tasty that will help you on your weight-loss journey:

Breakfast:

- Oatmeal with Berries and Almonds
1. Cook oats in water or milk (or, if you'd like, a dairy-free alternative).
2. Fresh berries like strawberries, blueberries, and raspberries should be added on top, along with a garnish of chopped almonds.
3. Add a little honey or maple syrup for sweetness.
- Avocado Toast
1. Toast whole-grain bread.
2. Spread mashed, ripe avocado on toast.
3. Sliced tomatoes, salt, pepper, and a dab of spicy sauce are added on top for flavor.

Lunch:

- Grilled Chicken Salad

1. Cook a chicken breast and cut it into slices.
2. Combine bell peppers, cherry tomatoes, cucumber slices, and mixed greens.
3. Use a low-calorie dressing of your choice or a light balsamic vinaigrette to coat the salad.
4. Add grilled chicken on top.
- Quinoa and Black Bean Bowl
1. After cooking the quinoa, combine it with the black beans, corn, tomatoes and cilantro.
2. Season the bowl with cumin, salt, and pepper after squeezing some fresh lime juice over it.
3. Add sliced avocado over top for richness.

Dinner:

- Baked Salmon with Steamed Broccoli
1. Garlic, lemon juice, and dill are used to season salmon fillets.
2. Bake in the oven until the salmon flakes with a fork without difficulty.
3. As a side, steam some fresh broccoli.

- Stir-Fried Tofu with Vegetables

1. Cut tofu into cubes and stir-fry it in a non-stick skillet with a variety of colorful veggies (such as bell peppers, snap peas, and carrots).

2. For flavor, mix in some low-sodium soy sauce or stir-fry sauce.

Snacks:

- Greek yogurt with sliced cucumber and fresh dill is a savory and filling snack.

- Mixed Nuts and Berries: Mix unsalted nuts (such as almonds, walnuts, and cashews) with dried berries (such as cranberries, and blueberries) to make a compact snack pack.